DIABETIC VEGAN COOKBOOKS FOR TYPE 2 DIABETES

Healthy Plant-Based Recipes for Managing Blood Sugar, Promoting Weight Loss, and Supporting Overall Wellness

By Mia Bennett

COPYRIGHT PAGE

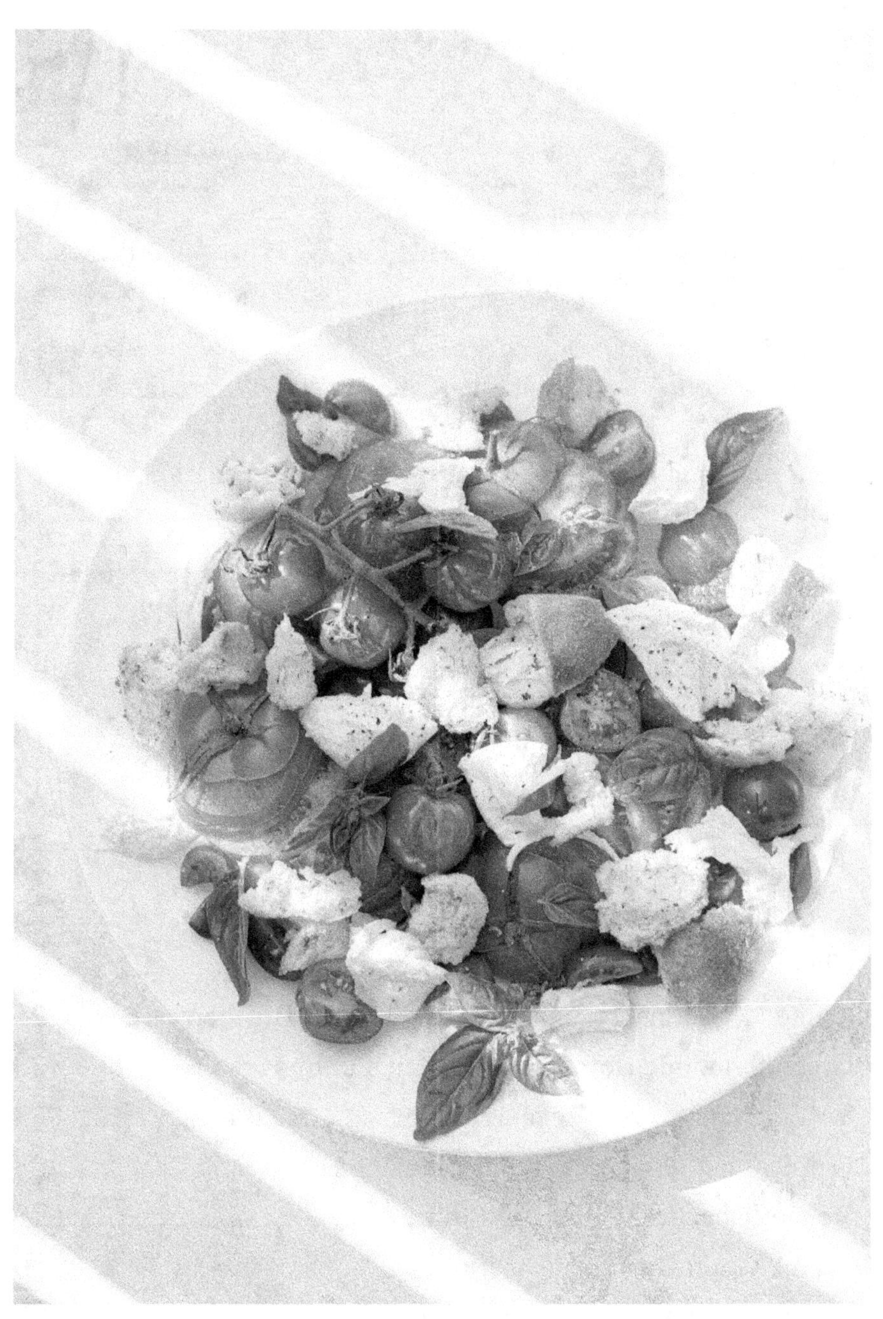

TABLE OF CONTENTS

Chapter 3: Lunch Recipes.. 38

Chapter 4: Dinner Recipes 55

Chapter 5: Snacks and Appetizers 77

INTRODUCTION

Imagine your body is a grand ball. Glucose, a type of sugar, is the fuel for the party, and insulin is the bouncer. In type 2 diabetes, the door gets sticky - insulin struggles to usher glucose into your cells for energy, causing a sugar build-up in the bloodstream. This imbalance can lead to long-term health issues.

The Vegan Advantage: Why Plants Can Be Powerful Allies

Here's where a vegan diet steps in as a potential game-changer. A well-planned vegan approach, rich in vegetables, fruits, whole grains, legumes, nuts, and seeds, offers a treasure trove of benefits:

- **Fiber Powerhouse:** Plant-based meals are naturally high in fiber, which slows down sugar absorption, promoting steadier blood sugar levels.
- **Weight Management:** Vegan diets often lead to healthy weight loss, which can significantly improve insulin sensitivity.
- **Bye-bye Bad Fats:** Saturated fats, common in animal products, can worsen insulin resistance. Plant-based fats tend to be healthier, supporting heart health.

Fueling Your Body Right: Nutritional Needs for Diabetic Vegans

While plants offer a bounty of goodness, some nutrients require extra attention on a vegan diabetic diet:

- **Protein**: Beans, lentils, tofu, tempeh, and nuts are your protein warriors. Aim for a variety to ensure you get all the essential amino acids.
- **Vitamin B12:** This crucial vitamin is mainly found in animal products. Fortified plant milks and nutritional yeast are excellent vegan sources. Consult your doctor to check your B12 levels and discuss supplementation if needed.
- **Omega-3 Fatty Acids:** These heart-healthy fats are abundant in fatty fish. Flaxseeds, chia seeds, and walnuts are fantastic vegan alternatives. Consider including them daily.

Building Your Vegan Diabetic Plate: Essential Ingredients and Substitutes

Here's your cheat sheet to stock your kitchen and conquer diabetes with plant-based power:

- **Protein Powerhouses:** Beans, lentils, tofu, tempeh, seitan, nuts, nut butter

- **Colorful Carbohydrates:** Whole grains (brown rice, quinoa), starchy vegetables (sweet potato, corn)
- **Fiber Fantastic Fruits**: Berries, apples, pears (all in moderation)
- **Healthy Fats:** Avocados, olives, nuts, seeds
- Sweet Alternatives: Spices like cinnamon and nutmeg can add sweetness without spiking blood sugar. Explore natural sweeteners like stevia in moderation.

Meal Planning and Prep: Mastering the Art of Delicious Diabetes Management

Conquering diabetes doesn't mean sacrificing flavor. Here are some tips for planning and prepping delicious, diabetic-friendly vegan meals:

- **Batch Cooking**: Cook a big pot of lentil soup or a quinoa stir-fry on the weekend for easy, grab-and-go lunches throughout the week.
- **Snack Savvy:** Stock up on pre-cut veggies, nuts, and fruits for healthy snacking. Hummus with veggie sticks makes a fantastic power-packed option.
- **Spice Up Your Life**: Experiment with herbs and spices to add variety and depth of flavor to your meals.

- **Read Food Labels:** Be mindful of hidden sugars and sodium in processed vegan foods. Opt for whole, unprocessed ingredients whenever possible.

Chapter 1: 30 Day Meal Plan

Week 1:

Day 1

- Breakfast: Avocado and Tomato Toast
- Lunch: Lentil and Vegetable Soup
- Dinner: Eggplant and Chickpea Tagine
- Snack: Roasted Chickpeas
- Dessert: Chia Seed Pudding with Mango

Day 2

- Breakfast: Chia Seed Pudding with Berries
- Lunch: Chickpea Salad Sandwich
- Dinner: Baked Tofu with Stir-Fried Vegetables
- Snack: Veggie Sticks with Hummus
- Dessert: Vegan Chocolate Avocado Mousse

Day 3

- Breakfast: Quinoa Breakfast Bowl with Almonds and Blueberries
- Lunch: Zucchini Noodles with Pesto
- Dinner: Lentil Shepherd's Pie
- Snack: Baked Kale Chips

- Dessert: Baked Cinnamon Apples

Day 4

- Breakfast: Green Smoothie Bowl with Spinach and Banana
- Lunch: Quinoa and Black Bean Salad
- Dinner: Vegan Jambalaya with Brown Rice
- Snack: Stuffed Mini Peppers with Guacamole
- Dessert: Almond Flour Blueberry Muffins

Day 5

- Breakfast: Tofu Scramble with Vegetables
- Lunch: Spinach and Mushroom Stuffed Peppers
- Dinner: Stuffed Acorn Squash with Quinoa and Cranberries
- Snack: Edamame with Sea Salt
- Dessert: Coconut Yogurt with Fresh Berries

Day 6

- Breakfast: Oatmeal with Flax Seeds and Cinnamon
- Lunch: Roasted Vegetable and Hummus Wrap
- Dinner: Cauliflower and Chickpea Tacos
- Snack: Vegan Spinach Artichoke Dip
- Dessert: Dark Chocolate and Nut Clusters

Day 7

- Breakfast: Vegan Pancakes with Fresh Fruit
- Lunch: Kale and Avocado Salad with Lemon Tahini Dressing
- Dinner: Vegan Pad Thai
- Snack: Cucumber and Avocado Sushi Bites
- Dessert: Vegan Banana Bread

Week 2:

Day 8

- Breakfast: Whole Grain Breakfast Burrito
- Lunch: Vegan Sushi Rolls
- Dinner: Mushroom and Spinach Lasagna
- Snack: Zucchini Fries with Vegan Ranch Dip
- Dessert: Raspberry Chia Jam Bars

Day 9

- Breakfast: Sweet Potato and Black Bean Hash
- Lunch: Grilled Portobello Mushroom Sandwich
- Dinner: Vegetable Paella
- Snack: Spicy Roasted Nuts
- Dessert: Mango Coconut Sorbet

Day 10

- Breakfast: Overnight Oats with Chia Seeds
- Lunch: Sweet Potato and Lentil Curry
- Dinner: Spicy Tempeh Chili
- Snack: Carrot and Beetroot Hummus
- Dessert: Raw Brownie Bites

Day 11

- Breakfast: Buckwheat Groats Porridge
- Lunch: Cauliflower Rice Stir-Fry
- Dinner: Roasted Brussels Sprouts and Sweet Potato Bowl
- Snack: Baked Sweet Potato Wedges
- Dessert: Vegan Lemon Cheesecake

Day 12

- Breakfast: Apple Cinnamon Quinoa Breakfast Bake
- Lunch: White Bean and Arugula Salad
- Dinner: Vegan Moussaka
- Snack: Vegan Stuffed Mushrooms
- Dessert: Apple Cinnamon Oat Bars

Day 13

- Breakfast: Peanut Butter and Banana Toast
- Lunch: Spaghetti Squash with Marinara Sauce

- Dinner: Thai Coconut Curry with Tofu
- Snack: Apple Slices with Almond Butter
- Dessert: Pumpkin Spice Cookies

Day 14

- Breakfast: Millet Porridge with Berries
- Lunch: Chickpea and Spinach Stew
- Dinner: Grilled Vegetable Kabobs with Quinoa
- Snack: Mini Vegan Quiches
- Dessert: Strawberry Coconut Macaroons

Week 3:

Day 15

- Breakfast: Carrot Cake Smoothie
- Lunch: Vegan Caesar Salad with Tofu Croutons
- Dinner: Butternut Squash and Sage Risotto
- Snack: Raw Energy Balls with Dates and Nuts
- Dessert: Chocolate-Dipped Fruit

Day 16

- Breakfast: Avocado and Tomato Toast
- Lunch: Lentil and Vegetable Soup
- Dinner: Eggplant and Chickpea Tagine

- Snack: Roasted Chickpeas
- Dessert: Chia Seed Pudding with Mango

Day 17

- Breakfast: Chia Seed Pudding with Berries
- Lunch: Chickpea Salad Sandwich
- Dinner: Baked Tofu with Stir-Fried Vegetables
- Snack: Veggie Sticks with Hummus
- Dessert: Vegan Chocolate Avocado Mousse

Day 18

- Breakfast: Quinoa Breakfast Bowl with Almonds and Blueberries
- Lunch: Zucchini Noodles with Pesto
- Dinner: Lentil Shepherd's Pie
- Snack: Baked Kale Chips
- Dessert: Baked Cinnamon Apples

Day 19

- Breakfast: Green Smoothie Bowl with Spinach and Banana
- Lunch: Quinoa and Black Bean Salad
- Dinner: Vegan Jambalaya with Brown Rice
- Snack: Stuffed Mini Peppers with Guacamole
- Dessert: Almond Flour Blueberry Muffins

Day 20

- Breakfast: Tofu Scramble with Vegetables
- Lunch: Spinach and Mushroom Stuffed Peppers
- Dinner: Stuffed Acorn Squash with Quinoa and Cranberries
- Snack: Edamame with Sea Salt
- Dessert: Coconut Yogurt with Fresh Berries

Day 21

- Breakfast: Oatmeal with Flax Seeds and Cinnamon
- Lunch: Roasted Vegetable and Hummus Wrap
- Dinner: Cauliflower and Chickpea Tacos
- Snack: Vegan Spinach Artichoke Dip
- Dessert: Dark Chocolate and Nut Clusters

Week 4:

Day 22

- Breakfast: Vegan Pancakes with Fresh Fruit
- Lunch: Kale and Avocado Salad with Lemon Tahini Dressing
- Dinner: Vegan Pad Thai
- Snack: Cucumber and Avocado Sushi Bites
- Dessert: Vegan Banana Bread

Day 23

- Breakfast: Whole Grain Breakfast Burrito
- Lunch: Vegan Sushi Rolls
- Dinner: Mushroom and Spinach Lasagna
- Snack: Zucchini Fries with Vegan Ranch Dip
- Dessert: Raspberry Chia Jam Bars

Day 24

- Breakfast: Sweet Potato and Black Bean Hash
- Lunch: Grilled Portobello Mushroom Sandwich
- Dinner: Vegetable Paella
- Snack: Spicy Roasted Nuts
- Dessert: Mango Coconut Sorbet

Day 25

- Breakfast: Overnight Oats with Chia Seeds
- Lunch: Sweet Potato and Lentil Curry
- Dinner: Spicy Tempeh Chili
- Snack: Carrot and Beetroot Hummus
- Dessert: Raw Brownie Bites

Day 26

- Breakfast: Buckwheat Groats Porridge
- Lunch: Cauliflower Rice Stir-Fry

- Dinner: Roasted Brussels Sprouts and Sweet Potato Bowl
- Snack: Baked Sweet Potato Wedges
- Dessert: Vegan Lemon Cheesecake

Day 27

- Breakfast: Apple Cinnamon Quinoa Breakfast Bake
- Lunch: White Bean and Arugula Salad
- Dinner: Vegan Moussaka
- Snack: Vegan Stuffed Mushrooms
- Dessert: Apple Cinnamon Oat Bars

Day 28

- Breakfast: Peanut Butter and Banana Toast
- Lunch: Spaghetti Squash with Marinara Sauce
- Dinner: Thai Coconut Curry with Tofu
- Snack: Apple Slices with Almond Butter
- Dessert: Pumpkin Spice Cookies

Day 29

- Breakfast: Millet Porridge with Berries
- Lunch: Chickpea and Spinach Stew
- Dinner: Grilled Vegetable Kabobs with Quinoa
- Snack: Mini Vegan Quiches
- Dessert: Strawberry Coconut Macaroons

Day 30

- Breakfast: Carrot Cake Smoothie
- Lunch: Vegan Caesar Salad with Tofu Croutons
- Dinner: Butternut Squash and Sage Risotto
- Snack: Raw Energy Balls with Dates and Nuts
- Dessert: Chocolate-Dipped Fruit

Chapter 2: Breakfast Recipes

Starting your day with a nutritious breakfast is essential for managing type 2 diabetes and maintaining overall health. The following vegan breakfast recipes are designed to be delicious, satisfying, and balanced to keep your blood sugar levels stable. Each recipe includes simple instructions and nutritional information to help you make informed choices.

Avocado and Tomato Toast

Ingredients:

- 1 ripe avocado
- 1 medium tomato, sliced
- 2 slices whole grain bread
- Salt and pepper to taste
- Lemon juice

Instructions:

1. Toast the bread slices.
2. Mash the avocado and spread it on the toast.
3. Top with tomato slices.
4. Season with salt, pepper, and a squeeze of lemon juice.

Nutrition Information (per serving):

- Calories: 250
- Protein: 6g
- Carbohydrates: 28g
- Fat: 14g
- Fiber: 10g
- Sugar: 3g
- Portion size: 2 slices

Chia Seed Pudding with Berries

Ingredients:

- 3 tbsp chia seeds
- 1 cup almond milk
- 1 tbsp maple syrup
- 1/2 cup mixed berries

Instructions:

1. Combine chia seeds, almond milk, and maple syrup in a bowl.
2. Stir well and refrigerate overnight.
3. Top with mixed berries before serving.

Nutrition Information (per serving):

- Calories: 200
- Protein: 5g
- Carbohydrates: 26g
- Fat: 9g
- Fiber: 12g
- Sugar: 10g
- Portion size: 1 cup

Quinoa Breakfast Bowl with Almonds and Blueberries

Ingredients:

- 1 cup cooked quinoa
- 1/4 cup almonds, chopped
- 1/2 cup fresh blueberries
- 1 tbsp maple syrup
- 1/2 cup almond milk

Instructions:

1. Place cooked quinoa in a bowl.
2. Top with almonds and blueberries.
3. Drizzle with maple syrup and almond milk.

Nutrition Information (per serving):

- Calories: 350
- Protein: 10g
- Carbohydrates: 48g
- Fat: 14g
- Fiber: 8g
- Sugar: 14g
- Portion size: 1 bowl

Green Smoothie Bowl with Spinach and Banana

Ingredients:

- 1 cup spinach
- 1 banana
- 1/2 cup almond milk
- 1 tbsp chia seeds
- 1/4 cup granola

Instructions:

1. Blend spinach, banana, and almond milk until smooth.
2. Pour into a bowl and top with chia seeds and granola.

Nutrition Information (per serving):

- Calories: 250
- Protein: 5g
- Carbohydrates: 42g
- Fat: 8g
- Fiber: 7g
- Sugar: 18g
- Portion size: 1 bowl

Tofu Scramble with Vegetables

Ingredients:

- 1 block firm tofu, crumbled
- 1 bell pepper, diced
- 1 onion, diced
- 1 tsp turmeric
- Salt and pepper to taste

Instructions:

1. Sauté onion and bell pepper until soft.
2. Add crumbled tofu and turmeric.
3. Cook for 5-7 minutes, seasoning with salt and pepper.

Nutrition Information (per serving):

- Calories: 200
- Protein: 14g
- Carbohydrates: 10g
- Fat: 12g
- Fiber: 4g
- Sugar: 3g
- Portion size: 1 cup

Oatmeal with Flax Seeds and Cinnamon

Ingredients:

- 1/2 cup rolled oats
- 1 cup water or almond milk
- 1 tbsp flax seeds
- 1 tsp cinnamon
- 1 tbsp maple syrup

Instructions:

1. Cook oats in water or almond milk according to package instructions.
2. Stir in flax seeds, cinnamon, and maple syrup.

Nutrition Information (per serving):

- Calories: 200
- Protein: 5g
- Carbohydrates: 35g
- Fat: 5g
- Fiber: 7g
- Sugar: 8g
- Portion size: 1 bowl

Vegan Pancakes with Fresh Fruit

Ingredients:

- 1 cup whole wheat flour
- 1 tbsp baking powder
- 1 cup almond milk
- 1 tbsp maple syrup
- Fresh fruit for topping

Instructions:

1. Mix flour, baking powder, almond milk, and maple syrup.
2. Cook pancakes on a hot griddle until bubbles form.
3. Serve with fresh fruit.

Nutrition Information (per serving):

- Calories: 300
- Protein: 8g
- Carbohydrates: 56g
- Fat: 6g
- Fiber: 8g
- Sugar: 12g
- Portion size: 3 pancakes

Whole Grain Breakfast Burrito

Ingredients:

- 1 whole grain tortilla
- 1/2 cup black beans
- 1/4 cup salsa
- 1/4 avocado, sliced
- 1/4 cup spinach

Instructions:

1. Warm the tortilla.
2. Fill with black beans, salsa, avocado, and spinach.
3. Roll up and serve.

Nutrition Information (per serving):

- Calories: 300
- Protein: 10g
- Carbohydrates: 45g
- Fat: 10g
- Fiber: 12g
- Sugar: 4g
- Portion size: 1 burrito

Sweet Potato and Black Bean Hash

Ingredients:

- 1 large sweet potato, diced
- 1/2 cup black beans
- 1/2 onion, diced
- 1 bell pepper, diced
- 1 tsp cumin

Instructions:

1. Sauté onion and bell pepper until soft.
2. Add sweet potato and cook until tender.
3. Stir in black beans and cumin, cooking until heated through.

Nutrition Information (per serving):

- Calories: 250
- Protein: 6g
- Carbohydrates: 45g
- Fat: 6g
- Fiber: 10g
- Sugar: 8g
- Portion size: 1 cup

Overnight Oats with Chia Seeds

Ingredients:

- 1/2 cup rolled oats
- 1 cup almond milk
- 1 tbsp chia seeds
- 1 tbsp maple syrup
- Fresh fruit for topping

Instructions:

1. Combine oats, almond milk, chia seeds, and maple syrup in a jar.
2. Refrigerate overnight.
3. Top with fresh fruit before serving.

Nutrition Information (per serving):

- Calories: 250
- Protein: 6g
- Carbohydrates: 42g
- Fat: 8g
- Fiber: 8g
- Sugar: 12g
- Portion size: 1 jar

Buckwheat Groats Porridge

Ingredients:

- 1/2 cup buckwheat groats
- 1 cup water or almond milk
- 1 tbsp maple syrup
- 1/2 cup fresh berries

Instructions:

1. Cook buckwheat groats in water or almond milk until tender.
2. Stir in maple syrup and top with berries.

Nutrition Information (per serving):

- Calories: 250
- Protein: 6g

- Carbohydrates: 46g

- Fat: 4g

- Fiber: 8g

- Sugar: 10g

- Portion size: 1 bowl

Apple Cinnamon Quinoa Breakfast Bake

Ingredients:

- 1 cup cooked quinoa

- 1 apple, diced

- 1 tsp cinnamon

- 1 tbsp maple syrup

- 1/4 cup almond milk

Instructions:

1. Preheat oven to 350°F.

2. Mix quinoa, apple, cinnamon, maple syrup, and almond milk.

3. Bake for 20 minutes.

Nutrition Information (per serving):

- Calories: 300

- Protein: 8g

- Carbohydrates: 58g

- Fat: 5g

- Fiber: 8g

- Sugar: 18g

- Portion size: 1 bowl

Peanut Butter and Banana Toast

Ingredients:

- 2 slices whole grain bread

- 2 tbsp peanut butter

- 1 banana, sliced

Instructions:

1. Toast the bread slices.

2. Spread peanut butter on the toast.

3. Top with banana slices.

Nutrition Information (per serving):

- Calories: 350

- Protein: 10g

- Carbohydrates: 45g

- Fat: 16g

- Fiber: 8g

- Sugar: 14g
- Portion size: 2 slices

Millet Porridge with Berries

Ingredients:

- 1/2 cup millet
- 1 cup water or almond milk
- 1 tbsp maple syrup
- 1/2 cup fresh berries

Instructions:

1. Cook millet in water or almond milk until tender.
2. Stir in maple syrup and top with berries.

Nutrition Information (per serving):

- Calories: 250
- Protein: 6g
- Carbohydrates: 46g
- Fat: 4g
- Fiber: 6g
- Sugar: 10g
- Portion size: 1 bowl

Carrot Cake Smoothie

Ingredients:

- 1 cup almond milk
- 1/2 cup carrots, grated
- 1 banana
- 1 tsp cinnamon
- 1 tbsp chia seeds

Instructions:

1. Blend all ingredients until smooth.
2. Serve immediately.

Nutrition Information (per serving):

- Calories: 200
- Protein: 4g
- Carbohydrates: 42g
- Fat: 4g
- Fiber: 7g
- Sugar: 22g
- Portion size: 1 smoothie

Chapter 3: Lunch Recipes

A healthy and satisfying lunch can make all the difference in maintaining energy levels and managing blood sugar throughout the day. These vegan lunch recipes are designed to be nutritious, delicious, and suitable for those managing Type 2 diabetes. Each recipe includes a balance of proteins, healthy fats, and fiber-rich carbohydrates to help you stay full and satisfied.

Lentil and Vegetable Soup

Ingredients:

- 1 cup dried lentils
- 1 carrot, diced
- 1 celery stalk, diced
- 1 onion, diced
- 2 garlic cloves, minced
- 4 cups vegetable broth
- 1 can diced tomatoes
- 1 tsp thyme
- Salt and pepper to taste

Instructions:

1. Rinse lentils and set aside.

2. In a large pot, sauté onion, carrot, celery, and garlic until softened.

3. Add lentils, vegetable broth, tomatoes, and thyme.

4. Bring to a boil, then reduce heat and simmer for 30 minutes.

5. Season with salt and pepper.

Nutrition Information (per serving, serves 4):

- Calories: 180
- Protein: 12g
- Carbohydrates: 30g
- Fat: 1g
- Fiber: 12g
- Sugar: 6g
- Portion Size: 1 cup

Chickpea Salad Sandwich

Ingredients:

- 1 can chickpeas, drained and mashed
- 2 tbsp vegan mayonnaise
- 1 celery stalk, diced
- 1 green onion, chopped
- 1 tsp Dijon mustard
- Salt and pepper to taste

- Whole grain bread
- Lettuce and tomato slices

Instructions:

1. Mix mashed chickpeas, vegan mayo, celery, green onion, and mustard.
2. Season with salt and pepper.
3. Spread on whole grain bread and top with lettuce and tomato.

Nutrition Information (per serving, serves 2):

- Calories: 350
- Protein: 12g
- Carbohydrates: 55g
- Fat: 10g
- Fiber: 12g
- Sugar: 6g
- Portion Size: 1 sandwich

Zucchini Noodles with Pesto

Ingredients:

- 2 large zucchinis, spiralized
- 1 cup fresh basil leaves

- 1/4 cup pine nuts

- 2 garlic cloves

- 1/4 cup olive oil

- 2 tbsp nutritional yeast

- Salt and pepper to taste

Instructions:

1. Blend basil, pine nuts, garlic, olive oil, nutritional yeast, salt, and pepper to make pesto.

2. Toss zucchini noodles with pesto until well coated.

Nutrition Information (per serving, serves 2):

- Calories: 250

- Protein: 6g

- Carbohydrates: 10g

- Fat: 22g

- Fiber: 3g

- Sugar: 6g

- Portion Size: 1.5 cups

Quinoa and Black Bean Salad

Ingredients:

- 1 cup cooked quinoa

- 1 can black beans, drained and rinsed
- 1 red bell pepper, diced
- 1/2 cup corn kernels
- 1/4 cup chopped cilantro
- Juice of 1 lime
- Salt and pepper to taste

Instructions:

1. Combine quinoa, black beans, bell pepper, corn, and cilantro in a bowl.
2. Add lime juice, salt, and pepper, and toss to combine.

Nutrition Information (per serving, serves 4):

- Calories: 220
- Protein: 8g
- Carbohydrates: 35g
- Fat: 4g
- Fiber: 9g
- Sugar: 3g
- Portion Size: 1 cup

Spinach and Mushroom Stuffed Peppers

Ingredients:

- 4 bell peppers, tops removed and seeded
- 2 cups spinach, chopped
- 1 cup mushrooms, diced
- 1 onion, diced
- 1/2 cup quinoa, cooked
- 2 garlic cloves, minced
- Salt and pepper to taste

Instructions:

1. Sauté onion, mushrooms, and garlic until soft.
2. Add spinach and cook until wilted.
3. Stir in cooked quinoa, salt, and pepper.
4. Stuff mixture into bell peppers and bake at 375°F for 25 minutes.

Nutrition Information (per serving, serves 4):

- Calories: 180
- Protein: 6g
- Carbohydrates: 32g
- Fat: 3g
- Fiber: 7g
- Sugar: 7g

- Portion Size: 1 stuffed pepper

Roasted Vegetable and Hummus Wrap

Ingredients:

- 1 cup mixed vegetables (e.g., zucchini, bell peppers, onions), roasted
- 1/2 cup hummus
- Whole grain wrap
- Handful of spinach leaves

Instructions:

1. Spread hummus on the wrap.
2. Add roasted vegetables and spinach leaves.
3. Roll up the wrap tightly.

Nutrition Information (per serving, serves 2):

- Calories: 320
- Protein: 8g
- Carbohydrates: 45g
- Fat: 12g
- Fiber: 8g
- Sugar: 4g
- Portion Size: 1 wrap

Kale and Avocado Salad with Lemon Tahini Dressing

Ingredients:

- 4 cups kale, chopped
- 1 avocado, diced
- 1/4 cup sunflower seeds
- 1 lemon, juiced
- 2 tbsp tahini
- Salt and pepper to taste

Instructions:

1. Massage kale with lemon juice and tahini.
2. Add avocado and sunflower seeds.
3. Season with salt and pepper.

Nutrition Information (per serving, serves 2):

- Calories: 280
- Protein: 7g
- Carbohydrates: 20g
- Fat: 22g
- Fiber: 10g
- Sugar: 2g
- Portion Size: 1.5 cups

Vegan Sushi Rolls

Ingredients:

- 1 cup sushi rice, cooked
- 1 avocado, sliced
- 1 cucumber, julienned
- 1 carrot, julienned
- Nori sheets
- Soy sauce for dipping

Instructions:

1. Spread sushi rice on nori sheet.
2. Add avocado, cucumber, and carrot.
3. Roll tightly and slice into pieces.

Nutrition Information (per serving, serves 4):

- Calories: 180
- Protein: 4g
- Carbohydrates: 34g
- Fat: 4g
- Fiber: 3g
- Sugar: 2g
- Portion Size: 4 pieces

Grilled Portobello Mushroom Sandwich

Ingredients:

- 4 portobello mushrooms
- 1 red onion, sliced
- 4 whole grain buns
- Lettuce leaves
- 1/4 cup vegan mayonnaise

Instructions:

1. Grill mushrooms and onions until tender.
2. Spread vegan mayo on buns.
3. Assemble sandwich with mushrooms, onions, and lettuce.

Nutrition Information (per serving, serves 4):

- Calories: 300
- Protein: 8g
- Carbohydrates: 45g
- Fat: 10g
- Fiber: 5g
- Sugar: 5g
- Portion Size: 1 sandwich

Sweet Potato and Lentil Curry

Ingredients:

- 1 cup lentils, cooked
- 2 sweet potatoes, diced
- 1 onion, diced
- 1 can coconut milk
- 2 tbsp curry powder
- Salt and pepper to taste

Instructions:

1. Sauté onion until soft.
2. Add sweet potatoes, lentils, coconut milk, and curry powder.
3. Simmer until sweet potatoes are tender.

Nutrition Information (per serving, serves 4):

- Calories: 350
- Protein: 12g
- Carbohydrates: 60g
- Fat: 10g
- Fiber: 15g
- Sugar: 10g
- Portion Size: 1 cup

Cauliflower Rice Stir-Fry

Ingredients:

- 4 cups cauliflower rice
- 1 bell pepper, diced
- 1 cup snap peas
- 1 carrot, julienned
- 2 tbsp soy sauce
- 1 tbsp sesame oil

Instructions:

1. Stir-fry vegetables in sesame oil until tender.
2. Add cauliflower rice and soy sauce.
3. Cook until heated through.

Nutrition Information (per serving, serves 4):

- Calories: 120
- Protein: 4g
- Carbohydrates: 15g
- Fat: 6g
- Fiber: 5g
- Sugar: 5g
- Portion Size: 1.5 cups

White Bean and Arugula Salad

Ingredients:

- 1 can (15 oz) white beans, drained and rinsed
- 2 cups arugula
- 1 cup cherry tomatoes, halved
- 1/4 cup red onion, thinly sliced
- 2 tbsp olive oil
- 1 tbsp balsamic vinegar
- Salt and pepper to taste

Instructions:

1. In a large bowl, combine white beans, arugula, cherry tomatoes, and red onion.
2. Drizzle olive oil and balsamic vinegar over the salad.
3. Season with salt and pepper, toss gently to combine.
4. Serve immediately.

Nutrition Information (per serving):

- Calories: 280
- Protein: 12g
- Carbohydrates: 35g
- Fat: 10g
- Fiber: 10g
- Sugar: 2g

- Portion size: 1 bowl

Spaghetti Squash with Marinara Sauce

Ingredients:

- 1 medium spaghetti squash
- 2 cups marinara sauce (store-bought or homemade)
- Fresh basil leaves for garnish
- Salt and pepper to taste

Instructions:

1. Preheat oven to 400°F (200°C).
2. Cut spaghetti squash in half lengthwise and scoop out the seeds.
3. Place squash halves cut side down on a baking sheet. Bake for 40-45 minutes, or until tender.
4. Scrape the flesh of the squash with a fork to create spaghetti-like strands.
5. Heat marinara sauce in a saucepan until warmed through.
6. Serve spaghetti squash topped with marinara sauce and garnish with fresh basil leaves.
7. Season with salt and pepper to taste.

Nutrition Information (per serving):

- Calories: 180
- Protein: 4g
- Carbohydrates: 40g
- Fat: 2g
- Fiber: 10g
- Sugar: 15g
- Portion size: 1 squash half

Chickpea and Spinach Stew

Ingredients:

- 1 can (15 oz) chickpeas, drained and rinsed
- 2 cups fresh spinach leaves
- 1 onion, chopped
- 2 cloves garlic, minced
- 1 tsp cumin powder
- 1/2 tsp paprika
- 3 cups vegetable broth
- Salt and pepper to taste

Instructions:

1. In a large pot, sauté onion and garlic until softened.

2. Add cumin powder and paprika, stir for 1 minute until fragrant.

3. Add chickpeas and vegetable broth, bring to a simmer.

4. Cook for 15-20 minutes, or until chickpeas are tender.

5. Stir in fresh spinach leaves and cook until wilted.

6. Season with salt and pepper to taste.

7. Serve hot.

Nutrition Information (per serving):

- Calories: 250
- Protein: 12g
- Carbohydrates: 45g
- Fat: 4g
- Fiber: 12g
- Sugar: 8g
- Portion size: 1 bowl

Vegan Caesar Salad with Tofu Croutons

Ingredients:

- 1 head romaine lettuce, chopped
- 1/2 cup cherry tomatoes, halved
- 1/4 cup vegan Caesar dressing
- 1/2 cup firm tofu, cubed

- 1 tbsp olive oil

- Salt and pepper to taste

Instructions:

1. Preheat oven to 400°F (200°C).

2. Toss cubed tofu with olive oil, salt, and pepper.

3. Spread tofu cubes on a baking sheet and bake for 20-25 minutes, or until golden and crispy.

4. In a large bowl, combine chopped romaine lettuce and cherry tomatoes.

5. Add vegan Caesar dressing and toss to coat evenly.

6. Top salad with tofu croutons before serving.

Nutrition Information (per serving):

- Calories: 220

- Protein: 10g

- Carbohydrates: 15g

- Fat: 15g

- Fiber: 5g

- Sugar: 3g

- Portion size: 1 bowl

Chapter 4: Dinner Recipes

In Chapter 4, we explore a delightful array of dinner recipes that are both nutritious and satisfying, perfect for anyone following a vegan diet or managing type 2 diabetes. Each recipe is crafted to highlight the flavors and textures of plant-based ingredients, ensuring a delicious dining experience while supporting your health goals.

Eggplant and Chickpea Tagine

Ingredients:

- 1 large eggplant, cubed
- 1 can chickpeas, drained and rinsed
- 1 onion, diced
- 2 garlic cloves, minced
- 1 tsp ground cumin
- 1 tsp ground coriander
- 1/2 tsp turmeric
- 1/2 tsp cinnamon
- 1 cup vegetable broth
- Salt and pepper to taste
- Fresh cilantro for garnish

Instructions:

1. In a large pot, sauté onion and garlic until translucent.

2. Add eggplant and spices, cook until eggplant begins to soften.

3. Stir in chickpeas and vegetable broth. Simmer for 20-25 minutes.

4. Season with salt and pepper. Serve hot, garnished with fresh cilantro.

Nutrition Information:

*   Calories: 320
*   Protein: 12g
*   Carbohydrates: 54g
*   Fat: 7g
*   Fiber: 14g
*   Sugar: 12g
*   Portion Size: 1 1/2 cups

Baked Tofu with Stir-Fried Vegetables

Ingredients:

*   1 block firm tofu, pressed and cubed
*   2 cups mixed vegetables (broccoli, bell peppers, snap peas)
*   2 tbsp soy sauce

- 1 tbsp maple syrup
- 1 tbsp sesame oil
- 1 tsp minced ginger
- 1 garlic clove, minced
- Salt and pepper to taste

Instructions:

1. Preheat oven to 400°F (200°C). Arrange tofu cubes on a baking sheet and bake for 25-30 minutes until golden.
2. In a pan, heat sesame oil and sauté ginger and garlic until fragrant.
3. Add mixed vegetables and stir-fry until tender-crisp.
4. Stir in baked tofu, soy sauce, and maple syrup. Cook for 2-3 minutes. Serve hot.

Nutrition Information:

- Calories: 280
- Protein: 18g
- Carbohydrates: 25g
- Fat: 12g
- Fiber: 6g
- Sugar: 10g
- Portion Size: 1 cup

Lentil Shepherd's Pie

Ingredients:

- 1 cup green lentils, cooked
- 2 carrots, diced
- 1 onion, diced
- 1 cup frozen peas
- 2 garlic cloves, minced
- 1 tbsp tomato paste
- 1 tsp dried thyme
- 1 tsp dried rosemary
- 2 cups mashed potatoes (prepared separately)
- Salt and pepper to taste

Instructions:

1. Preheat oven to 375°F (190°C). In a pan, sauté onion and garlic until softened.
2. Add carrots and cook for 5 minutes. Stir in cooked lentils, peas, tomato paste, and herbs.
3. Season with salt and pepper. Transfer mixture to a baking dish.
4. Spread mashed potatoes evenly over the lentil mixture. Bake for 25-30 minutes until golden.

Nutrition Information:

- Calories: 350
- Protein: 15g
- Carbohydrates: 60g
- Fat: 5g
- Fiber: 15g
- Sugar: 8g
- Portion Size: 1 cup

Vegan Jambalaya with Brown Rice

Ingredients:

- 1 cup brown rice, cooked
- 1 onion, diced
- 1 bell pepper, diced
- 2 celery stalks, diced
- 1 can diced tomatoes
- 1 can kidney beans, drained and rinsed
- 1 cup vegetable broth
- 1 tsp paprika
- 1/2 tsp dried thyme
- 1/2 tsp dried oregano
- Salt and pepper to taste
- Hot sauce (optional)

Instructions:

1. In a large skillet, sauté onion, bell pepper, and celery until softened.

2. Stir in diced tomatoes, kidney beans, vegetable broth, and spices. Simmer for 15-20 minutes.

3. Fold in cooked brown rice and cook for an additional 5 minutes until heated through.

4. Season with salt, pepper, and hot sauce if desired. Serve hot.

Nutrition Information:

- Calories: 300
- Protein: 12g
- Carbohydrates: 55g
- Fat: 2g
- Fiber: 12g
- Sugar: 8g
- Portion Size: 1 cup

Stuffed Acorn Squash with Quinoa and Cranberries

Ingredients:

- 2 acorn squashes, halved and seeded
- 1 cup quinoa, cooked

- 1/2 cup dried cranberries
- 1/4 cup chopped pecans
- 1 tbsp maple syrup
- 1 tsp cinnamon
- Salt and pepper to taste

Instructions:

1. Preheat oven to 400°F (200°C). Place acorn squash halves on a baking sheet, cut side down. Bake for 30-35 minutes until tender.
2. In a bowl, combine cooked quinoa, cranberries, pecans, maple syrup, cinnamon, salt, and pepper.
3. Fill each squash half with quinoa mixture. Return to oven and bake for an additional 10 minutes.
4. Serve hot, garnished with additional pecans if desired.

Nutrition Information:

- Calories: 320
- Protein: 8g
- Carbohydrates: 60g
- Fat: 7g
- Fiber: 10g
- Sugar: 15g
- Portion Size: 1 stuffed half squash

Cauliflower and Chickpea Tacos

Ingredients:

- 1 small head cauliflower, cut into florets
- 1 can chickpeas, drained and rinsed
- 1 tbsp olive oil
- 1 tsp chili powder
- 1/2 tsp cumin
- 1/2 tsp smoked paprika
- Salt and pepper to taste
- 8 small corn tortillas
- Toppings: avocado, salsa, cilantro

Instructions:

1. Preheat oven to 400°F (200°C). Toss cauliflower florets and chickpeas with olive oil, chili powder, cumin, smoked paprika, salt, and pepper.
2. Spread on a baking sheet and roast for 20-25 minutes until cauliflower is tender and chickpeas are crispy.
3. Warm corn tortillas in a dry skillet or microwave.
4. Assemble tacos with roasted cauliflower and chickpeas. Top with avocado, salsa, and cilantro. Serve warm.

Nutrition Information:

- Calories: 250

- Protein: 8g
- Carbohydrates: 40g
- Fat: 8g
- Fiber: 10g
- Sugar: 3g
- Portion Size: 2 tacos

Vegan Pad Thai

Ingredients:

- 8 oz rice noodles, cooked according to package instructions
- 1 cup tofu, cubed
- 1 cup bean sprouts
- 1 carrot, julienned
- 1 bell pepper, thinly sliced
- 1/2 cup chopped green onions
- 1/4 cup chopped peanuts
- Sauce: 1/4 cup soy sauce, 2 tbsp lime juice, 2 tbsp maple syrup, 1 tbsp rice vinegar, 1 tsp sriracha

Instructions:

1. In a large skillet, stir-fry tofu until golden brown. Add carrot, bell pepper, and green onions. Cook until vegetables are tender-crisp.

2. Add cooked rice noodles and bean sprouts to the skillet. Pour sauce over the noodles and toss until well combined.

3. Cook for 2-3 minutes until heated through. Serve hot, garnished with chopped peanuts.

Nutrition Information:

- Calories: 380
- Protein: 15g
- Carbohydrates: 60g
- Fat: 10g
- Fiber: 6g
- Sugar: 12g
- Portion Size: 1 1/2 cups

Mushroom and Spinach Lasagna

Ingredients:

- 9 lasagna noodles, cooked according to package instructions
- 2 cups sliced mushrooms (cremini or button)
- 3 cups baby spinach
- 2 cloves garlic, minced
- 2 cups marinara sauce
- 1 cup vegan ricotta cheese
- 1/2 cup vegan mozzarella cheese, shredded

- Salt and pepper to taste
- Fresh basil for garnish

Instructions:

1. Preheat oven to 375°F (190°C). In a pan, sauté mushrooms and garlic until mushrooms are tender.
2. Add baby spinach and cook until wilted. Season with salt and pepper.
3. Spread a thin layer of marinara sauce on the bottom of a baking dish. Layer with lasagna noodles, mushroom-spinach mixture, and dollops of vegan ricotta cheese.
4. Repeat layers, ending with a layer of marinara sauce. Sprinkle vegan mozzarella cheese on top.
5. Cover with foil and bake for 30 minutes. Remove foil and bake for an additional 10 minutes until cheese is melted and bubbly.
6. Let cool slightly before serving. Garnish with fresh basil.

Nutrition Information:

- Calories: 380
- Protein: 15g
- Carbohydrates: 55g
- Fat: 12g
- Fiber: 8g

- Sugar: 10g
- Portion Size: 1/6th of lasagna

Vegetable Paella

Ingredients:

- 1 cup Arborio rice
- 2 cups vegetable broth
- 1 onion, diced
- 2 garlic cloves, minced
- 1 red bell pepper, sliced
- 1 cup green beans, trimmed
- 1 cup artichoke hearts, quartered
- 1/2 cup frozen peas
- 1 tsp smoked paprika
- 1/2 tsp saffron threads (optional)
- Salt and pepper to taste
- Lemon wedges for serving

Instructions:

1. In a large skillet, sauté onion and garlic until softened. Add red bell pepper and cook for 2-3 minutes.
2. Stir in Arborio rice, smoked paprika, and saffron threads. Cook for 1 minute.

3. Pour vegetable broth into the skillet. Bring to a simmer and cook, stirring occasionally, until rice is almost tender, about 15 minutes.

4. Add green beans, artichoke hearts, and peas. Cook for an additional 5-7 minutes until vegetables are tender and rice is fully cooked.

5. Season with salt and pepper. Serve hot with lemon wedges.

Nutrition Information:

- Calories: 320
- Protein: 8g
- Carbohydrates: 65g
- Fat: 3g
- Fiber: 8g
- Sugar: 5g
- Portion Size: 1 cup

Spicy Tempeh Chili

Ingredients:

- 8 oz tempeh, crumbled
- 1 onion, diced
- 2 garlic cloves, minced
- 1 bell pepper, diced

- 1 can kidney beans, drained and rinsed
- 1 can diced tomatoes
- 2 cups vegetable broth
- 1 tbsp chili powder
- 1 tsp cumin
- 1/2 tsp smoked paprika
- Salt and pepper to taste
- Fresh cilantro for garnish

Instructions:

1. In a large pot, sauté onion and garlic until softened.
2. Add crumbled tempeh, bell pepper, chili powder, cumin, and smoked paprika. Cook for 5-7 minutes until tempeh is lightly browned.
3. Stir in kidney beans, diced tomatoes, and vegetable broth. Bring to a boil, then reduce heat and simmer for 20-25 minutes.
4. Season with salt and pepper. Serve hot, garnished with fresh cilantro.

Nutrition Information:

- Calories: 300
- Protein: 20g
- Carbohydrates: 35g

- Fat: 10g
- Fiber: 12g
- Sugar: 8g
- Portion Size: 1 1/2 cups

Roasted Brussels Sprouts and Sweet Potato Bowl

Ingredients:

- 2 cups Brussels sprouts, halved
- 2 cups sweet potatoes, diced
- 1 tbsp olive oil
- 1 tsp smoked paprika
- 1/2 tsp garlic powder
- Salt and pepper to taste
- 1 cup quinoa, cooked
- 1/4 cup tahini dressing (tahini, lemon juice, water, salt)

Instructions:

1. Preheat oven to 400°F (200°C). Toss Brussels sprouts and sweet potatoes with olive oil, smoked paprika, garlic powder, salt, and pepper.
2. Spread on a baking sheet and roast for 25-30 minutes until vegetables are tender and caramelized.

3. Divide cooked quinoa into bowls. Top with roasted Brussels sprouts and sweet potatoes.

4. Drizzle with tahini dressing. Serve warm.

Nutrition Information:

- Calories: 380

- Protein: 12g

- Carbohydrates: 60g

- Fat: 12g

- Fiber: 12g

- Sugar: 8g

- Portion Size: 1 bowl

Vegan Moussaka

Ingredients:

- 2 medium eggplants, sliced lengthwise

- 1 cup lentils, cooked

- 1 onion, diced

- 2 garlic cloves, minced

- 1 can diced tomatoes

- 1/2 cup tomato sauce

- 1 tsp dried oregano

- 1 tsp dried basil

- Salt and pepper to taste
- 1 cup vegan béchamel sauce (made with plant-based milk and flour)
- Fresh parsley for garnish

Instructions:

1. Preheat oven to 375°F (190°C). Brush eggplant slices with olive oil and arrange on a baking sheet. Bake for 20 minutes until softened.
2. In a pan, sauté onion and garlic until translucent. Add cooked lentils, diced tomatoes, tomato sauce, oregano, basil, salt, and pepper. Simmer for 10 minutes.
3. Layer half of the eggplant slices in a baking dish. Spread half of the lentil mixture on top. Repeat with remaining eggplant and lentil mixture.
4. Pour vegan béchamel sauce evenly over the top layer. Bake for 30-35 minutes until golden and bubbly.
5. Let cool slightly before serving. Garnish with fresh parsley.

Nutrition Information:

- Calories: 350
- Protein: 15g
- Carbohydrates: 50g
- Fat: 10g

- Fiber: 12g

- Sugar: 10g

- Portion Size: 1/6th of moussaka

Thai Coconut Curry with Tofu

Ingredients:

- 1 block tofu, cubed

- 1 onion, diced

- 1 bell pepper, sliced

- 1 zucchini, sliced

- 1 cup snap peas

- 1 can coconut milk

- 2 tbsp Thai red curry paste

- 1 tbsp soy sauce

- 1 tbsp maple syrup

- Juice of 1 lime

- Fresh cilantro for garnish

Instructions:

1. In a large skillet, sauté tofu cubes until golden brown. Remove from skillet and set aside.

2. In the same skillet, sauté onion, bell pepper, zucchini, and snap peas until tender.

3. Stir in coconut milk, Thai red curry paste, soy sauce, maple syrup, and lime juice. Simmer for 10 minutes.

4. Add tofu back to the skillet and cook for an additional 5 minutes.

5. Serve hot, garnished with fresh cilantro. Serve over rice or noodles if desired.

Nutrition Information:

- Calories: 400
- Protein: 20g
- Carbohydrates: 25g
- Fat: 25g
- Fiber: 8g
- Sugar: 10g
- Portion Size: 1 1/2 cups

Grilled Vegetable Kabobs with Quinoa

Ingredients:

- 1 zucchini, sliced into rounds
- 1 yellow bell pepper, cut into chunks
- 1 red onion, cut into chunks
- 1 cup cherry tomatoes
- 8 oz mushrooms, whole

- 1/4 cup olive oil
- 2 tbsp balsamic vinegar
- 1 tsp dried thyme
- Salt and pepper to taste
- 1 cup quinoa, cooked

Instructions:

1. In a bowl, combine olive oil, balsamic vinegar, dried thyme, salt, and pepper.
2. Thread zucchini rounds, bell pepper chunks, red onion chunks, cherry tomatoes, and mushrooms onto skewers.
3. Brush vegetable kabobs with the olive oil mixture.
4. Grill over medium-high heat for 10-12 minutes, turning occasionally, until vegetables are tender and lightly charred.
5. Serve grilled vegetable kabobs over cooked quinoa. Drizzle with any remaining olive oil mixture. Serve hot.

Nutrition Information:

- Calories: 320
- Protein: 10g
- Carbohydrates: 40g
- Fat: 15g
- Fiber: 8g
- Sugar: 8g

- Portion Size: 1 kabob skewer with quinoa

Butternut Squash and Sage Risotto

Ingredients:

- 1 butternut squash, peeled, seeded, and diced
- 1 onion, diced
- 2 garlic cloves, minced
- 1 1/2 cups Arborio rice
- 1/2 cup white wine (optional)
- 4 cups vegetable broth, heated
- 1 tbsp fresh sage leaves, chopped
- 1/4 cup nutritional yeast (optional)
- Salt and pepper to taste

Instructions:

1. In a large pot, sauté onion and garlic until softened.
2. Add diced butternut squash and Arborio rice. Stir to coat rice with oil.
3. If using, pour in white wine and cook until wine is absorbed.
4. Gradually add hot vegetable broth, one ladleful at a time, stirring frequently and allowing each addition to be absorbed before adding the next.
5. Cook until rice is creamy and tender, about 20-25 minutes.

6. Stir in chopped sage leaves and nutritional yeast. Season with salt and pepper.

7. Remove from heat and let rest for a few minutes before serving.

Nutrition Information:

- Calories: 380
- Protein: 8g
- Carbohydrates: 75g
- Fat: 5g
- Fiber: 8g
- Sugar: 8g
- Portion Size: 1 cup

Chapter 5: Snacks and Appetizers

Snacking can be both delicious and nutritious, especially for those managing diabetes with a vegan diet. These snacks and appetizers are designed to satisfy cravings while providing essential nutrients. From crunchy kale chips to creamy hummus dips, each recipe offers a balance of flavors and textures to keep you energized throughout the day.

Roasted Chickpeas

Ingredients:

- 1 can (15 oz) chickpeas, drained and rinsed
- 1 tablespoon olive oil
- 1 teaspoon smoked paprika
- 1/2 teaspoon garlic powder
- Salt to taste

Instructions:

1. Preheat oven to 400°F (200°C).
2. Pat dry chickpeas with a towel to remove excess moisture.
3. Toss chickpeas with olive oil, smoked paprika, garlic powder, and salt.
4. Spread chickpeas in a single layer on a baking sheet.

5. Roast for 25-30 minutes until crispy, shaking the pan halfway through.

6. Let cool before serving.

Nutrition Information (per serving):

- Calories: 150

- Protein: 6g

- Carbohydrates: 22g

- Fat: 5g

- Fiber: 6g

- Sugar: 4g

- Serving Size: 1/2 cup

Veggie Sticks with Hummus

Ingredients:

- Carrot sticks, cucumber sticks, bell pepper strips

- 1 cup homemade or store-bought hummus

Instructions:

1. Wash and cut vegetables into sticks or strips.

2. Serve with hummus for dipping.

Nutrition Information (per serving):

- Calories: 120
- Protein: 5g
- Carbohydrates: 15g
- Fat: 6g
- Fiber: 7g
- Sugar: 3g
- Serving Size: 1 cup of vegetables with 2 tablespoons hummus

Baked Kale Chips

Ingredients:

- 1 bunch kale, washed and dried thoroughly
- 1 tablespoon olive oil
- Salt to taste

Instructions:

1. Preheat oven to 275°F (135°C).
2. Remove kale leaves from stems and tear into bite-sized pieces.
3. Massage kale with olive oil and sprinkle with salt.
4. Spread kale in a single layer on a baking sheet.

5. Bake for 20-25 minutes until crispy, rotating the pan halfway through.

6. Let cool before serving.

Nutrition Information (per serving):

- Calories: 80
- Protein: 5g
- Carbohydrates: 8g
- Fat: 4g
- Fiber: 2g
- Sugar: 1g
- Serving Size: 1 cup

Stuffed Mini Peppers with Guacamole

Ingredients:

- Mini sweet peppers, halved and deseeded
- 2 ripe avocados
- 1 lime, juiced
- Salt and pepper to taste
- Optional: chopped cilantro, diced tomatoes

Instructions:

1. Scoop avocado flesh into a bowl and mash with lime juice, salt, and pepper.
2. Stir in optional ingredients if desired.
3. Spoon guacamole into halved mini peppers.
4. Serve immediately or chill before serving.

Nutrition Information (per serving):

- Calories: 100
- Protein: 2g
- Carbohydrates: 7g
- Fat: 8g
- Fiber: 4g
- Sugar: 2g
- Serving Size: 4 stuffed mini peppers

Edamame with Sea Salt

Ingredients:

- 1 cup frozen edamame, thawed
- Sea salt to taste

Instructions:

1. Steam or microwave edamame according to package instructions.

2. Sprinkle with sea salt before serving.

Nutrition Information (per serving):

- Calories: 120

- Protein: 11g

- Carbohydrates: 9g

- Fat: 4g

- Fiber: 8g

- Sugar: 2g

- Serving Size: 1 cup

Vegan Spinach Artichoke Dip

Ingredients:

- 1 cup raw cashews, soaked in water for 2 hours, drained

- 1 cup cooked spinach, squeezed dry

- 1 can (14 oz) artichoke hearts, drained and chopped

- 1/4 cup nutritional yeast

- 1/4 cup unsweetened almond milk

- 2 cloves garlic, minced

- Salt and pepper to taste

Instructions:

1. Blend soaked cashews, almond milk, nutritional yeast, and garlic until smooth.
2. Stir in spinach and chopped artichoke hearts.
3. Season with salt and pepper.
4. Serve warm or chilled with veggie sticks or whole grain crackers.

Nutrition Information (per serving):

- Calories: 180
- Protein: 9g
- Carbohydrates: 15g
- Fat: 10g
- Fiber: 6g
- Sugar: 2g
- Serving Size: 1/4 cup

Cucumber and Avocado Sushi Bites

Ingredients:

- 1 cucumber, cut into thick slices
- 1 ripe avocado, thinly sliced
- Nori seaweed sheets, cut into strips
- Soy sauce or tamari, for serving (optional)

- Pickled ginger and wasabi, for serving (optional)

Instructions:

1. Place a slice of cucumber on a serving dish.
2. Top with a slice of avocado and a strip of nori seaweed.
3. Repeat for remaining cucumber slices.
4. Serve with soy sauce, pickled ginger, and wasabi if desired.

Nutrition Information (per serving):

- Calories: 80
- Protein: 2g
- Carbohydrates: 6g
- Fat: 6g
- Fiber: 4g
- Sugar: 1g
- Serving Size: 4 pieces

Zucchini Fries with Vegan Ranch Dip

Ingredients:

- 2 zucchinis, cut into fries
- 1/2 cup breadcrumbs (gluten-free if desired)
- 1/4 cup nutritional yeast
- 1 teaspoon garlic powder

- Salt and pepper to taste
- Vegan ranch dip for serving

Instructions:

1. Preheat oven to 425°F (220°C) and line a baking sheet with parchment paper.
2. In a bowl, mix breadcrumbs, nutritional yeast, garlic powder, salt, and pepper.
3. Coat zucchini fries in the breadcrumb mixture and place on the baking sheet.
4. Bake for 20-25 minutes until crispy, flipping halfway through.
5. Serve with vegan ranch dip.

Nutrition Information (per serving):

- Calories: 150
- Protein: 5g
- Carbohydrates: 25g
- Fat: 3g
- Fiber: 5g
- Sugar: 5g
- Serving Size: 1 zucchini (about 10 fries) with dip

Spicy Roasted Nuts

Ingredients:

- 2 cups mixed raw nuts (such as almonds, cashews, walnuts)
- 1 tablespoon olive oil
- 1 teaspoon smoked paprika
- 1/2 teaspoon cayenne pepper
- Salt to taste

Instructions:

1. Preheat oven to 350°F (175°C).
2. Toss nuts with olive oil, smoked paprika, cayenne pepper, and salt.
3. Spread nuts in a single layer on a baking sheet.
4. Roast for 10-12 minutes, stirring halfway through.
5. Let cool before serving.

Nutrition Information (per serving):

- Calories: 200
- Protein: 7g
- Carbohydrates: 8g
- Fat: 17g
- Fiber: 4g
- Sugar: 2g
- Serving Size: 1/4 cup

Carrot and Beetroot Hummus

Ingredients:

- 1 cup cooked chickpeas
- 1 medium carrot, peeled and chopped
- 1 small beetroot, peeled and chopped
- 2 tablespoons tahini
- Juice of 1 lemon
- 1 clove garlic, minced
- Salt and pepper to taste
- Water (as needed to adjust consistency)

Instructions:

1. In a food processor, blend cooked chickpeas, carrot, beetroot, tahini, lemon juice, garlic, salt, and pepper until smooth.
2. Add water gradually if needed to reach desired consistency.
3. Adjust seasoning to taste.
4. Serve with vegetable sticks or whole grain crackers.

Nutrition Information (per serving):

- Calories: 120
- Protein: 5g
- Carbohydrates: 15g
- Fat: 5g

- Fiber: 4g
- Sugar: 3g
- Serving Size: 1/4 cup

Baked Sweet Potato Wedges

Ingredients:

- 2 medium sweet potatoes, scrubbed and cut into wedges
- 1 tablespoon olive oil
- 1 teaspoon smoked paprika
- 1/2 teaspoon garlic powder
- Salt and pepper to taste

Instructions:

1. Preheat oven to 425°F (220°C) and line a baking sheet with parchment paper.
2. In a bowl, toss sweet potato wedges with olive oil, smoked paprika, garlic powder, salt, and pepper.
3. Arrange wedges in a single layer on the baking sheet.
4. Bake for 25-30 minutes, flipping halfway through, until golden and crispy.
5. Serve warm.

Nutrition Information (per serving):

- Calories: 150
- Protein: 2g
- Carbohydrates: 26g
- Fat: 4g
- Fiber: 4g
- Sugar: 5g
- Serving Size: 1 medium sweet potato (about 8 wedges)

Vegan Stuffed Mushrooms

Ingredients:

- 12 large button mushrooms, stems removed and finely chopped
- 1/2 cup breadcrumbs (gluten-free if desired)
- 1/4 cup chopped fresh parsley
- 1/4 cup nutritional yeast
- 2 tablespoons olive oil
- 2 cloves garlic, minced
- Salt and pepper to taste

Instructions:

1. Preheat oven to 375°F (190°C) and line a baking sheet with parchment paper.

2. In a bowl, combine chopped mushroom stems, breadcrumbs, parsley, nutritional yeast, olive oil, garlic, salt, and pepper.

3. Spoon mixture into mushroom caps, pressing gently to fill.

4. Arrange stuffed mushrooms on the baking sheet.

5. Bake for 20-25 minutes until mushrooms are tender and golden.

6. Serve warm.

Nutrition Information (per serving):

- Calories: 120

- Protein: 5g

- Carbohydrates: 15g

- Fat: 5g

- Fiber: 3g

- Sugar: 3g

- Serving Size: 3 stuffed mushrooms

Apple Slices with Almond Butter

Ingredients:

- 1 apple, sliced

- 2 tablespoons almond butter

- Optional: sprinkle of cinnamon

Instructions:

1. Slice the apple into thin wedges.

2. Spread almond butter on each apple slice.

3. Sprinkle with cinnamon if desired.

4. Serve immediately.

Nutrition Information (per serving):

- Calories: 150

- Protein: 3g

- Carbohydrates: 20g

- Fat: 8g

- Fiber: 5g

- Sugar: 13g

- Serving Size: 1 medium apple with almond butter

Mini Vegan Quiches

Ingredients:

- 1 cup chickpea flour

- 1 cup unsweetened almond milk

- 1/2 cup diced vegetables (such as bell peppers, spinach, tomatoes)

- 1/4 cup nutritional yeast

- 1 teaspoon baking powder

- 1/2 teaspoon turmeric
- Salt and pepper to taste

Instructions:

1. Preheat oven to 375°F (190°C) and grease a mini muffin tin.
2. In a bowl, whisk chickpea flour, almond milk, nutritional yeast, baking powder, turmeric, salt, and pepper until smooth.
3. Stir in diced vegetables.
4. Pour mixture into the muffin tin, filling each cup 3/4 full.
5. Bake for 20-25 minutes until set and lightly golden.
6. Let cool before removing from tin.

Nutrition Information (per serving, 2 mini quiches):

- Calories: 120
- Protein: 7g
- Carbohydrates: 15g
- Fat: 4g
- Fiber: 3g
- Sugar: 2g
- Serving Size: 2 mini quiches

Raw Energy Balls with Dates and Nuts

Ingredients:

- 1 cup pitted dates
- 1 cup mixed nuts (such as almonds, cashews, walnuts)
- 1/4 cup unsweetened shredded coconut
- 1 tablespoon chia seeds
- 1 tablespoon cocoa powder
- Pinch of salt

Instructions:

1. In a food processor, blend dates and nuts until finely chopped and sticky.
2. Add shredded coconut, chia seeds, cocoa powder, and salt. Pulse until combined.
3. Roll mixture into small balls using hands.
4. Optional: Roll balls in additional coconut or cocoa powder.
5. Chill in the refrigerator for 30 minutes before serving.

Nutrition Information (per serving, 2 balls):

- Calories: 150
- Protein: 4g
- Carbohydrates: 20g
- Fat: 8g
- Fiber: 4g

- Sugar: 14g
- Serving Size: 2 energy balls

Chapter 6: Desserts

Indulging in delicious desserts while maintaining a diabetic-friendly vegan diet is entirely possible with these creative and wholesome recipes. Each dessert not only satisfies your sweet cravings but also provides essential nutrients without spiking your blood sugar levels. From fruity delights to rich chocolate treats, these recipes are designed to be both flavorful and health-conscious.

Chia Seed Pudding with Mango

Ingredients:

- 1/4 cup chia seeds
- 1 cup unsweetened almond milk
- 1 tablespoon maple syrup (optional)
- 1/2 teaspoon vanilla extract
- 1 ripe mango, diced

Instructions:

1. In a bowl, mix chia seeds, almond milk, maple syrup (if using), and vanilla extract. Stir well.
2. Let it sit for 10 minutes, then stir again to prevent clumping.
3. Cover and refrigerate overnight or for at least 4 hours until it thickens.

4. Serve chilled, topped with diced mango.

Nutrition Information (per serving):

- Calories: 220
- Protein: 5g
- Carbohydrates: 32g
- Fat: 8g
- Fiber: 10g
- Sugar: 18g
- Portion size: 1 cup

Vegan Chocolate Avocado Mousse

Ingredients:

- 2 ripe avocados
- 1/4 cup cocoa powder
- 1/4 cup maple syrup
- 1 teaspoon vanilla extract
- Fresh berries for garnish (optional)

Instructions:

1. Scoop the flesh of avocados into a food processor.
2. Add cocoa powder, maple syrup, and vanilla extract. Blend until smooth and creamy.

3. Transfer to serving bowls and refrigerate for 1 hour.

4. Garnish with fresh berries before serving.

Nutrition Information (per serving):

- Calories: 180
- Protein: 3g
- Carbohydrates: 21g
- Fat: 11g
- Fiber: 7g
- Sugar: 10g
- Portion size: 1/2 cup

Baked Cinnamon Apples

Ingredients:

- 4 medium apples, cored and sliced
- 1 tablespoon coconut oil, melted
- 1 teaspoon ground cinnamon
- 1 tablespoon maple syrup (optional)
- 1/4 cup chopped nuts (walnuts or almonds)

Instructions:

1. Preheat the oven to 350°F (175°C).

2. In a bowl, toss apple slices with melted coconut oil, cinnamon, and maple syrup (if using), ensuring they are evenly coated.

3. Spread the apples in a baking dish and bake for 20-25 minutes, until tender.

4. Sprinkle with chopped nuts before serving.

Nutrition Information (per serving):

- Calories: 160
- Protein: 2g
- Carbohydrates: 26g
- Fat: 7g
- Fiber: 6g
- Sugar: 18g
- Portion size: 1 apple equivalent

Almond Flour Blueberry Muffins

Ingredients:

- 2 cups almond flour
- 1/2 teaspoon baking soda
- 1/4 teaspoon salt
- 1/4 cup maple syrup
- 1/4 cup unsweetened applesauce

- 2 tablespoons coconut oil, melted
- 1 teaspoon vanilla extract
- 1 cup fresh or frozen blueberries

Instructions:

1. Preheat the oven to 350°F (175°C). Line a muffin tin with paper liners.
2. In a large bowl, mix almond flour, baking soda, and salt.
3. In another bowl, whisk together maple syrup, applesauce, coconut oil, and vanilla extract.
4. Combine wet and dry ingredients, then gently fold in blueberries.
5. Spoon batter into muffin cups, filling each about 3/4 full.
6. Bake for 20-25 minutes, until a toothpick inserted into the center comes out clean.
7. Allow muffins to cool before serving.

Nutrition Information (per muffin):

- Calories: 180
- Protein: 5g
- Carbohydrates: 14g
- Fat: 12g
- Fiber: 3g
- Sugar: 8g

- Portion size: 1 muffin

Coconut Yogurt with Fresh Berries

Ingredients:

- 1 cup unsweetened coconut yogurt
- 1 cup mixed fresh berries (such as strawberries, blueberries, raspberries)

Instructions:

1. Spoon coconut yogurt into serving bowls.
2. Top with mixed fresh berries.
3. Serve immediately.

Nutrition Information (per serving):

- Calories: 120
- Protein: 2g
- Carbohydrates: 15g
- Fat: 6g
- Fiber: 3g
- Sugar: 10g
- Portion size: 1 cup

Dark Chocolate and Nut Clusters

Ingredients:

- 1/2 cup dark chocolate chips (70% cocoa or higher)
- 1/2 cup mixed nuts (almonds, cashews, walnuts), chopped

Instructions:

1. Melt dark chocolate chips in a microwave-safe bowl in 30-second intervals, stirring in between until smooth.
2. Stir in chopped nuts until well combined.
3. Drop spoonfuls of the mixture onto a parchment-lined baking sheet.
4. Refrigerate for 30 minutes, or until chocolate is set.
5. Enjoy as a delicious treat.

Nutrition Information (per serving, approximately 2 clusters):

- Calories: 150
- Protein: 3g
- Carbohydrates: 12g
- Fat: 10g
- Fiber: 3g
- Sugar: 7g
- Portion size: 2 clusters

Vegan Banana Bread

Ingredients:

- 3 ripe bananas, mashed
- 1/4 cup coconut oil, melted
- 1/2 cup maple syrup
- 1 teaspoon vanilla extract
- 1 3/4 cups whole wheat flour
- 1 teaspoon baking powder
- 1/2 teaspoon baking soda
- 1/2 teaspoon salt
- 1/2 cup chopped walnuts (optional)

Instructions:

1. Preheat the oven to 350°F (175°C). Grease a loaf pan or line with parchment paper.
2. In a large bowl, mix mashed bananas, melted coconut oil, maple syrup, and vanilla extract.
3. In another bowl, whisk together whole wheat flour, baking powder, baking soda, and salt.
4. Combine wet and dry ingredients until just combined. Fold in chopped walnuts, if using.
5. Pour batter into the prepared loaf pan.
6. Bake for 50-60 minutes, or until a toothpick inserted into the center comes out clean.

7. Allow banana bread to cool in the pan for 10 minutes before transferring to a wire rack to cool completely.

Nutrition Information (per slice, assuming 12 slices per loaf):

- Calories: 220
- Protein: 4g
- Carbohydrates: 32g
- Fat: 9g
- Fiber: 3g
- Sugar: 14g
- Portion size: 1 slice

Raspberry Chia Jam Bars

Ingredients:

- 1 cup rolled oats
- 1/2 cup almond flour
- 1/4 cup coconut oil, melted
- 1/4 cup maple syrup
- 1/2 cup raspberry chia jam (store-bought or homemade)

Instructions:

1. Preheat the oven to 350°F (175°C). Line an 8x8 inch baking pan with parchment paper.

2. In a bowl, combine rolled oats, almond flour, melted coconut oil, and maple syrup. Mix until crumbly.

3. Press half of the oat mixture evenly into the bottom of the prepared pan.

4. Spread raspberry chia jam over the oat layer.

5. Sprinkle the remaining oat mixture evenly over the jam layer and press gently.

6. Bake for 25-30 minutes, or until the top is golden brown.

7. Allow to cool completely in the pan before cutting into bars.

Nutrition Information (per bar, assuming 12 bars):

- Calories: 160
- Protein: 3g
- Carbohydrates: 20g
- Fat: 8g
- Fiber: 3g
- Sugar: 8g
- Portion size: 1 bar

Mango Coconut Sorbet

Ingredients:

- 2 cups frozen mango chunks
- 1/2 cup coconut milk

- 1 tablespoon maple syrup (optional)
- Fresh mint leaves for garnish (optional)

Instructions:

1. In a blender or food processor, blend frozen mango chunks, coconut milk, and maple syrup (if using) until smooth and creamy.
2. Serve immediately for a soft-serve consistency, or transfer to a container and freeze for 1-2 hours for a firmer sorbet.
3. Garnish with fresh mint leaves before serving.

Nutrition Information (per serving):

- Calories: 150
- Protein: 1g
- Carbohydrates: 30g
- Fat: 5g
- Fiber: 3g
- Sugar: 25g
- Portion size: 1/2 cup

Raw Brownie Bites

Ingredients:

- 1 cup walnuts

- 1 cup pitted dates
- 3 tablespoons cocoa powder
- 1/2 teaspoon vanilla extract
- Pinch of salt
- Unsweetened shredded coconut for rolling (optional)

Instructions:

1. In a food processor, blend walnuts until finely ground.
2. Add pitted dates, cocoa powder, vanilla extract, and salt. Process until mixture sticks together.
3. Roll the mixture into small balls, about 1 inch in diameter.
4. Optionally, roll each ball in shredded coconut to coat.
5. Refrigerate for at least 30 minutes before serving.

Nutrition Information (per bite, assuming 16 bites):

- Calories: 90
- Protein: 2g
- Carbohydrates: 12g
- Fat: 5g
- Fiber: 2g
- Sugar: 9g
- Portion size: 1 bite

Vegan Lemon Cheesecake

Ingredients:

- 1 1/2 cups raw cashews, soaked overnight
- 1/4 cup coconut oil, melted
- 1/4 cup maple syrup
- Zest and juice of 2 lemons
- 1 teaspoon vanilla extract
- 1/2 cup coconut cream (from a chilled can of full-fat coconut milk)
- 1/2 cup shredded coconut for crust (optional)

Instructions:

1. Line a 9-inch round cake pan with parchment paper or use a springform pan.
2. In a food processor, blend soaked cashews, melted coconut oil, maple syrup, lemon zest and juice, and vanilla extract until smooth.
3. In a separate bowl, whip coconut cream until fluffy, then fold into the cashew mixture.
4. Pour mixture into the prepared pan and smooth the top with a spatula.
5. Optionally, sprinkle shredded coconut over the top for a crust-like texture.
6. Refrigerate for at least 4 hours, or until set.

7. Slice and serve chilled.

Nutrition Information (per slice, assuming 10 slices):

- Calories: 280
- Protein: 5g
- Carbohydrates: 20g
- Fat: 22g
- Fiber: 2g
- Sugar: 10g
- Portion size: 1 slice

Apple Cinnamon Oat Bars

Ingredients:

- 2 cups rolled oats
- 1/2 cup almond flour
- 1 teaspoon ground cinnamon
- 1/2 teaspoon baking powder
- 1/4 teaspoon salt
- 1/2 cup unsweetened applesauce
- 1/4 cup maple syrup
- 1/4 cup coconut oil, melted
- 1 teaspoon vanilla extract
- 2 medium apples, peeled and diced

Instructions:

1. Preheat the oven to 350°F (175°C). Grease an 8x8 inch baking pan or line with parchment paper.
2. In a large bowl, mix rolled oats, almond flour, ground cinnamon, baking powder, and salt.
3. In another bowl, whisk together applesauce, maple syrup, melted coconut oil, and vanilla extract.
4. Combine wet and dry ingredients until well incorporated. Fold in diced apples.
5. Press the mixture evenly into the prepared baking pan.
6. Bake for 30-35 minutes, or until lightly golden brown.
7. Allow to cool completely in the pan before cutting into bars.

Nutrition Information (per bar, assuming 12 bars):

- Calories: 180
- Protein: 4g
- Carbohydrates: 24g
- Fat: 8g
- Fiber: 3g
- Sugar: 10g
- Portion size: 1 bar

Pumpkin Spice Cookies

Ingredients:

- 1 cup canned pumpkin puree
- 1/4 cup coconut oil, melted
- 1/2 cup maple syrup
- 1 teaspoon vanilla extract
- 2 cups whole wheat flour
- 1 teaspoon baking powder
- 1/2 teaspoon baking soda
- 1 teaspoon ground cinnamon
- 1/2 teaspoon ground ginger
- 1/4 teaspoon ground nutmeg
- 1/4 teaspoon ground cloves
- 1/4 teaspoon salt

Instructions:

1. Preheat the oven to 350°F (175°C). Line a baking sheet with parchment paper.
2. In a large bowl, mix pumpkin puree, melted coconut oil, maple syrup, and vanilla extract.
3. In another bowl, whisk together whole wheat flour, baking powder, baking soda, spices, and salt.
4. Combine wet and dry ingredients until well combined.

5. Drop spoonfuls of dough onto the prepared baking sheet, spacing them about 2 inches apart.

6. Flatten each cookie slightly with the back of a spoon.

7. Bake for 12-15 minutes, or until cookies are firm and lightly golden.

8. Allow to cool on the baking sheet for 5 minutes before transferring to a wire rack to cool completely.

Nutrition Information (per cookie, assuming 24 cookies):

- Calories: 90
- Protein: 2g
- Carbohydrates: 14g
- Fat: 3g
- Fiber: 2g
- Sugar: 5g
- Portion size: 1 cookie

Strawberry Coconut Macaroons

Ingredients:

- 3 cups shredded coconut, unsweetened
- 1/2 cup coconut flour
- 1/2 cup coconut milk
- 1/4 cup maple syrup

- 1 teaspoon vanilla extract
- 1/2 cup chopped fresh strawberries

Instructions:

1. Preheat the oven to 325°F (160°C). Line a baking sheet with parchment paper.
2. In a large bowl, combine shredded coconut and coconut flour.
3. In a separate bowl, whisk together coconut milk, maple syrup, and vanilla extract.
4. Pour the wet ingredients over the dry ingredients and mix until well combined.
5. Fold in chopped strawberries gently.
6. Scoop tablespoon-sized portions of the mixture onto the prepared baking sheet, pressing each mound together firmly.
7. Bake for 20-25 minutes, or until the edges are golden brown.
8. Allow to cool on the baking sheet for 10 minutes before transferring to a wire rack to cool completely.

Nutrition Information (per macaroon, assuming 24 macaroons):

- Calories: 110
- Protein: 1g
- Carbohydrates: 10g
- Fat: 7g

- Fiber: 3g
- Sugar: 6g
- Portion size: 1 macaroon

Chocolate-Dipped Fruit

Ingredients:

- Assorted fresh fruit (such as strawberries, banana slices, pineapple chunks)
- 1/2 cup dark chocolate chips (70% cocoa or higher)

Instructions:

1. Line a baking sheet with parchment paper.
2. Wash and dry the fresh fruit thoroughly.
3. Melt dark chocolate chips in a microwave-safe bowl in 30-second intervals, stirring until smooth.
4. Dip each piece of fruit halfway into the melted chocolate, allowing any excess chocolate to drip off.
5. Place the chocolate-dipped fruit onto the prepared baking sheet.
6. Refrigerate for 10-15 minutes, or until the chocolate is set.
7. Serve chilled.

Nutrition Information (per serving, assuming 1/2 cup of mixed fruit):

- Calories: 150
- Protein: 2g
- Carbohydrates: 25g
- Fat: 6g
- Fiber: 5g
- Sugar: 18g
- Portion size: 1/2 cup

Chapter 7: Smoothies

Smoothies are a refreshing and nutritious way to start your day or boost your energy levels. Packed with vitamins, minerals, and antioxidants, these recipes offer a delicious blend of flavors while supporting your health goals. Whether you're looking for a green detox option or a tropical delight, these smoothies are designed to satisfy and nourish.

Green Detox Smoothie

Ingredients:

- 1 cup spinach
- 1/2 cucumber, peeled and chopped
- 1/2 green apple, chopped
- 1/2 lemon, juiced
- 1/2 inch fresh ginger, grated
- 1 cup coconut water or water
- Ice cubes (optional)

Instructions:

1. Combine all ingredients in a blender.
2. Blend until smooth.
3. Serve immediately.

Nutrition Information:

- Calories: 90
- Protein: 2g
- Carbohydrates: 21g
- Fat: 0.5g
- Fiber: 5g
- Sugar: 12g
- Portion size: 1 serving

Berry Blast Smoothie

Ingredients:

- 1 cup mixed berries (strawberries, blueberries, raspberries)
- 1/2 banana
- 1/2 cup plain Greek yogurt (or dairy-free yogurt)
- 1 tbsp honey or maple syrup (optional)
- 1/2 cup almond milk or other milk of choice
- Ice cubes (optional)

Instructions:

1. Combine berries, banana, yogurt, honey (if using), and almond milk in a blender.
2. Blend until smooth.
3. Add ice cubes if desired and blend again until smooth.

Nutrition Information:

- Calories: 180
- Protein: 8g
- Carbohydrates: 33g
- Fat: 3g
- Fiber: 6g
- Sugar: 23g
- Portion size: 1 serving

Tropical Mango Smoothie

Ingredients:

- 1 cup frozen mango chunks
- 1/2 cup pineapple chunks
- 1/2 banana
- 1/2 cup coconut milk
- 1/4 cup orange juice
- Ice cubes (optional)

Instructions:

1. Place mango, pineapple, banana, coconut milk, and orange juice in a blender.
2. Blend until smooth.
3. Add ice cubes if desired and blend again until smooth.

Nutrition Information:

- Calories: 220
- Protein: 2g
- Carbohydrates: 47g
- Fat: 5g
- Fiber: 5g
- Sugar: 36g
- Portion size: 1 serving

Peanut Butter Banana Smoothie

Ingredients:

- 1 banana
- 2 tbsp natural peanut butter
- 1 cup almond milk or other milk of choice
- 1 tbsp honey or maple syrup (optional)
- Ice cubes (optional)

Instructions:

1. Place banana, peanut butter, almond milk, and honey (if using) in a blender.
2. Blend until smooth.
3. Add ice cubes if desired and blend again until smooth.

Nutrition Information:

- Calories: 300
- Protein: 9g
- Carbohydrates: 34g
- Fat: 16g
- Fiber: 5g
- Sugar: 19g
- Portion size: 1 serving

Chocolate Spinach Smoothie

Ingredients:

- 1 cup fresh spinach
- 1 tbsp unsweetened cocoa powder
- 1/2 banana
- 1 cup almond milk or other milk of choice
- 1 tbsp honey or maple syrup (optional)
- Ice cubes (optional)

Instructions:

1. Blend spinach, cocoa powder, banana, almond milk, and honey (if using) until smooth.
2. Add ice cubes if desired and blend again until smooth.

Nutrition Information:

- Calories: 150
- Protein: 5g
- Carbohydrates: 27g
- Fat: 4g
- Fiber: 6g
- Sugar: 15g
- Portion size: 1 serving

Anti-Inflammatory Turmeric Smoothie

Ingredients:

- 1/2 cup frozen pineapple chunks
- 1/2 cup frozen mango chunks
- 1/2 tsp ground turmeric
- 1/2 tsp ground ginger
- 1 tbsp chia seeds
- 1 cup coconut water or water
- Ice cubes (optional)

Instructions:

1. Blend pineapple, mango, turmeric, ginger, chia seeds, and coconut water until smooth.
2. Add ice cubes if desired and blend again until smooth.

Nutrition Information:

- Calories: 180
- Protein: 4g
- Carbohydrates: 34g
- Fat: 4g
- Fiber: 8g
- Sugar: 22g
- Portion size: 1 serving

Mixed Berry and Chia Seed Smoothie

Ingredients:

- 1 cup mixed berries (strawberries, blueberries, raspberries)
- 1 tbsp chia seeds
- 1/2 cup spinach leaves
- 1/2 cup plain Greek yogurt (or dairy-free yogurt)
- 1/2 cup almond milk or other milk of choice
- Ice cubes (optional)

Instructions:

1. Blend berries, chia seeds, spinach, yogurt, and almond milk until smooth.
2. Add ice cubes if desired and blend again until smooth.

Nutrition Information:

- Calories: 200
- Protein: 10g
- Carbohydrates: 32g
- Fat: 4g
- Fiber: 9g
- Sugar: 18g
- Portion size: 1 serving

Creamy Avocado Smoothie

Ingredients:

- 1/2 ripe avocado
- 1/2 cup spinach leaves
- 1/2 cup cucumber, peeled and chopped
- 1/2 cup pineapple chunks
- Juice of 1/2 lime
- 1 cup coconut water or water
- Ice cubes (optional)

Instructions:

1. Blend avocado, spinach, cucumber, pineapple, lime juice, and coconut water until smooth.
2. Add ice cubes if desired and blend again until smooth.

Nutrition Information:

- Calories: 180
- Protein: 4g
- Carbohydrates: 27g
- Fat: 8g
- Fiber: 9g
- Sugar: 14g
- Portion size: 1 serving

Orange Carrot Ginger Smoothie

Ingredients:

- 1 large carrot, peeled and chopped
- Juice of 2 oranges
- 1/2 inch fresh ginger, grated
- 1/2 cup plain Greek yogurt (or dairy-free yogurt)
- 1/2 cup almond milk or other milk of choice
- Ice cubes (optional)

Instructions:

1. Blend carrot, orange juice, ginger, yogurt, and almond milk until smooth.
2. Add ice cubes if desired and blend again until smooth.

Nutrition Information:

- Calories: 160
- Protein: 8g
- Carbohydrates: 30g
- Fat: 2g
- Fiber: 5g
- Sugar: 20g
- Portion size: 1 serving

Kiwi and Kale Smoothie

Ingredients:

- 2 kiwis, peeled and chopped
- 1 cup kale leaves, stems removed
- 1/2 banana
- 1/2 cup coconut water or water
- Juice of 1/2 lime
- Ice cubes (optional)

Instructions:

1. Blend kiwis, kale, banana, coconut water, and lime juice until smooth.
2. Add ice cubes if desired and blend again until smooth.

Nutrition Information:

- Calories: 150
- Protein: 5g
- Carbohydrates: 35g
- Fat: 1g
- Fiber: 7g
- Sugar: 20g
- Portion size: 1 serving

Pineapple Coconut Smoothie

Ingredients:

- 1 cup frozen pineapple chunks
- 1/2 cup coconut milk
- 1/2 cup plain Greek yogurt (or dairy-free yogurt)
- 1 tbsp honey or maple syrup (optional)
- Ice cubes (optional)

Instructions:

1. Blend pineapple, coconut milk, yogurt, and honey (if using) until smooth.
2. Add ice cubes if desired and blend again until smooth.

Nutrition Information:

- Calories: 220
- Protein: 8g
- Carbohydrates: 38g
- Fat: 6g
- Fiber: 3g
- Sugar: 30g
- Portion size: 1 serving

Watermelon Mint Smoothie

Ingredients:

- 2 cups cubed seedless watermelon
- 1/4 cup fresh mint leaves
- Juice of 1/2 lime
- 1/2 cup coconut water or water
- Ice cubes (optional)

Instructions:

1. Blend watermelon, mint leaves, lime juice, and coconut water until smooth.
2. Add ice cubes if desired and blend again until smooth.

Nutrition Information:

- Calories: 80
- Protein: 1g
- Carbohydrates: 20g
- Fat: 0.5g
- Fiber: 1g
- Sugar: 17g
- Portion size: 1 serving

Blueberry Almond Milk Smoothie

Ingredients:

- 1 cup frozen blueberries
- 1 cup almond milk
- 1/2 banana
- 1 tbsp almond butter
- 1 tbsp honey or maple syrup (optional)
- Ice cubes (optional)

Instructions:

1. Blend blueberries, almond milk, banana, almond butter, and honey (if using) until smooth.
2. Add ice cubes if desired and blend again until smooth.

Nutrition Information:

- Calories: 250
- Protein: 5g
- Carbohydrates: 40g
- Fat: 9g
- Fiber: 8g
- Sugar: 26g
- Portion size: 1 serving

Pomegranate Power Smoothie

Ingredients:

- 1/2 cup pomegranate seeds
- 1/2 cup frozen strawberries
- 1/2 cup plain Greek yogurt (or dairy-free yogurt)
- 1/2 cup almond milk or other milk of choice
- 1 tbsp honey or maple syrup (optional)
- Ice cubes (optional)

Instructions:

1. Blend pomegranate seeds, strawberries, yogurt, almond milk, and honey (if using) until smooth.
2. Add ice cubes if desired and blend again until smooth.

Nutrition Information:

- Calories: 200
- Protein: 10g
- Carbohydrates: 35g
- Fat: 3g
- Fiber: 7g
- Sugar: 25g
- Portion size: 1 serving

Matcha Green Tea Smoothie

Ingredients:

- 1 tsp matcha green tea powder
- 1/2 cup frozen mango chunks
- 1/2 banana
- 1/2 cup coconut milk
- 1/2 cup spinach leaves
- Ice cubes (optional)

Instructions:

1. Blend matcha powder, mango, banana, coconut milk, and spinach until smooth.
2. Add ice cubes if desired and blend again until smooth.

Nutrition Information:

- Calories: 180
- Protein: 4g
- Carbohydrates: 30g
- Fat: 6g
- Fiber: 5g
- Sugar: 20g
- Portion size: 1 serving

CONCLUSION

Congratulations on completing your journey through the "Diabetic Vegan Cookbooks for Type 2 Diabetes"! This book has been crafted with your health and well-being in mind, offering a diverse array of delicious and nutritious recipes tailored specifically for managing type 2 diabetes through a vegan lifestyle.

Throughout this cookbook, you've explored innovative ways to create satisfying meals that prioritize plant-based ingredients while adhering to diabetic dietary guidelines. From hearty breakfasts to wholesome dinners, energizing smoothies to guilt-free desserts, each recipe has been thoughtfully curated to balance flavor, nutrition, and ease of preparation.

By embracing this cookbook, you've not only discovered new culinary delights but also empowered yourself with knowledge about managing diabetes through diet. You've learned about the benefits of veganism for diabetes, essential nutrients to incorporate, and practical tips for meal planning and preparation.

As you move forward, continue to explore and experiment with these recipes, adapting them to suit your preferences and lifestyle. Remember, maintaining a healthy diet is a journey, and each mindful choice contributes to your overall well-being. Stay committed to nourishing your body with wholesome, plant-based foods, and enjoy the journey to better health.

Thank you for choosing "Diabetic Vegan Cookbooks for Type 2 Diabetes". May your culinary adventures continue to inspire and support you on your path to a vibrant and fulfilling life. Here's to good health and delicious meals ahead!